KETO SMOOTHIE RECIPES

Introduction

I

have managed my weight for all intents and purposes for what seems like forever, since my teen years. I've been on a careful nutritional plan given that I was 15. I was consistently ravenous; I didn't have a phenomenal night's rest and energy for my everyday errands and

activities.

Quickly from that point forward, I stalled out in a pattern of "yo-yo consuming less calories" or weight gain, trailed by weight reduction. I contributed numerous years feeling wild with my eating. I felt like I was separated from my own body, and I didn't pay attention to it; be that as it may, I can't help myself. As a youngster of 17, I battled with anxiety.

I felt crushed; my buddies couldn't understand how this straight-An understudy and stunning lady may have any psychological issues. Additionally, my mothers and fathers failed to see what I was going through; they accepted I went through a stage like different teenagers with various feelings.

Later, when I stayed in school, my fights proceeded. I was abstaining from excessive food intake, once in a while actually in some cases not. It looks like a hamster on its wheel!

When I completed school, I had anything that I accepted I needed. All things considered, I wasn't really glad. I had a basically phobic concern of food, particularly oily food, nuts, and greasy cheese.

This conviction about fats depends on a well known fact that we have heard so often, so we assume it is valid. It resembles numerous different thoughts that fall into the classification of "misinterpretations" that are completely off-base! Incidentally, quality food, comprising of regular fats, is great for the human body.

In principle, assuming you wish to thin down, you should consume a greater number of calories than you eat; you should similarly consider routine activities, use the stairwell rather than lifts, walk an extra 30 minutes every day, blah, blah, blah. More straightforward expressed than done. By and by, we ought to analyze various components to understand that there is regularly more than one justification for weight gain. Mental elements, hereditary inclination, food dependence, high insulin levels, hormonal specialist unevenness, and neurologic issues all might play a part.

When I audit my life, I see low confidence and hopelessness. I likewise believed that cooking in your house is extended, Anyway I consistently bought food conveyance. I chose to quit mishandling myself and break the starve-gorge cycle. I decided to be more than happy! "Everything in your life is an impression of a choice you have made. Assuming you want a different result, make different choices," expressed Anonymous. So, I asked myself, "What causes you to feel relentlessly starving, notwithstanding eating satisfactory food and three dinners per day? How are you treating your body!? How would it be advisable for you treat you need to feel and put your best self forward?" These inquiries were convoluted for me, however somewhere down in my heart, I comprehended that the responses were simple. Fortunately, I tracked down the reactions and recuperate my relationship with food.

Among the main deterrents, I face while on the Ketogenic Diet is eating between suppers. This is explicitly genuine while at first start! Before our bodies begin involving fat as its essential wellspring of energy, our appetite levels are at its most noteworthy. That is the reason it's fundamental to have sound options to our typical undesirable impulses.

The Ketogenic amicable Fruit Drinks in this book are largely speedy and simple to make. You can drink them immediately, or store them somewhere cold to have while you're working. In any case, they will assist with keeping you full until your next meal.

The book is separated into two areas. The main half is loaded up with supplement thick beverages that are intended to provide your body with a shock of nutrients and minerals. The other half comprises of delectable Ketoaccommodating bite drinks. Consider these beverages little treats to praise yourself for adhering to the diet!

Thank you for perusing the book. Assuming you have any inquiries or remarks, I couldn't want anything more than to hear them!

A QUICK INTRODUCTION of the Ketogenic Diet regimen

Have you at any point before wished to have much more energy in your day, truly feel better as well as look better? Many individuals have found a way to accomplish a superior existence with a direct eating regimen plan. I comprehend it additionally appears to be incredible to be valid. However, it is feasible to get more power, truly feel far superior as well as look much better by changing the means you eat. There is no enchanted tablet; all things being equal, it is just about as straightforward as creating an eating plan that offers your body the supplements it needs.

What is this magic consuming plan ?

It is known as a Ketogenic Diet. This methodology of consuming isn't really new and has been around for endless years. Notwithstanding, contemporary society is picking cheap food, commonly stacked with carbs, and furthermore further developed sugars. Today, consuming is done on the run.

Comfort markets, as well as producers, satisfy clients' requests. These cheap food incorporate synthetic compounds, colors, added refined sugar, salt, and furthermore refined grains. While it could be helpful to our timetable, these food varieties are not issue free for our body to process.

The Ketogenic Diet might appear to be innovative as well as convoluted, yet essentially, this diet plan is taking care of your body food sources that it can refine all the more advantageously. The body is made to work involving nourishment for gas, which thus offers us power. The Ketogenic Diet upgrades this cycle with the aftereffect of giving us more energy. There are four assets of fuel for the body: sugars, fat, protein, and ketones.

But what are ketones? Ketones happen when fat in the body is separated. The consequence of a Ketogenic Diet is that fat and ketones become the essential wellspring of fuel for the body. The way to eating a Ketogenic Diet is to consume more fats, some protein, and little carbs. This permits the body to be in a condition of healthful ketosis.

Before beginning any sort of diet routine, you expect to examine the advantages/chances with your PCP. It is vital to perceive the impact an eating regimen plan might have on your body and furthermore your clinical issues. This will without a doubt assist you with picking an eating routine arrangement that will be protected and offer ideal results.

Eating a Ketogenic Diet isn't simply eating a low sugar diet. Rather than counting carbs, consider monitoring your body and how it is reacting to the food sources you eat. Is it true that you are giving yourself the supplements that you want? A Ketogenic Diet is an adjustment of both way of life and mindset.

When the body utilizes carbs to change glucose over to energy, glucose levels can drop quick. The outcomes are appetite and longings for sugar and carbs. On a Ketogenic Diet, drops in glucose are limited. This is on the grounds that fats and ketones fill in as fuel rather than speedy consuming carbs. Weight reduction is ruined by food sources that cause longings for sugar, salt, and fats. These habit-forming food varieties cause overconsumption of food that never gives a genuine sensation of fulfillment. Most frequently, handled food sources are the guilty parties. On a Ketogenic Diet, these food sources can be kept away from, as are the subsequent lousy nourishment desires and counting, stick to food sources found in pronounce.

appetite. Rather than calorie nature and that are easy to

Foods like grains, dairy, and furthermore cleaned sugar reason expanding in the body. Irritation prevents weight reduction and makes poisons develop in your body. In the wake of beginning the Ketogenic Diet, the poisons will be taken out, and expanding will decrease.

Enjoy your total smoothie formula below.

Part One

Delightful Nutritious Smoothies

hese plans are supplement thick creations that will top you off and move you along over the course of the day. These shakes are really great for you as well as taste incredible too!

Avocado-Blueberry Fruit Drink

his Fruit Drink isn't green, so even children will cherish it. The avocado makes the consistency of the Fruit Drink creamier and more rich. The blueberries load it with fiber and cancer prevention agent, which helps ward off free extremists and coronary illness.. I observe that even without the additional sugar, the blueberries improve the Fruit Drink enough.

Ingredients:
- 1/4 cup frozen blueberries, unsweetened
- 1/4 avocado, stripped, pitted, sliced
- 1/2 cup unsweetened almond milk, vanilla
- 1 scoop vanilla seclude protein or 2 tablespoons gelatin
- 1 tablespoon weighty cream
- 1 pack Stevia or 2 teaspoons Splenda

Instructions:
Put everything in a blender. Mix for until smooth. Pour in a glass.

Enjoy!

Serves: 2
Prep. Time: 4 minutes
Blend Time: 3 minutes
Dietetic Facts
Serving Size: 219
g Calories: 227
Total Fat: 14.6 g
Saturated Fat: 3.9 g Trans. Fat: 0 g
Cholesterol: 10 mg
Sodium: 124 mg
Potassium: 362 mg
Total Carbohydrates: 13 g
Dietary Fiber: 4.2 g Sugar: 6.2 g
Protein: 13.8 g

Vitamin A: 3% Calcium: 16% Vitamin C: 14%
Iron: 8%

Energizing Fruit Drink

N

ot just is this thick Fruit Drink flavorful, yet the cranberries additionally load it with against bacterial properties that assist with forestalling kidney ulcers. Cranberry juice is also perceived to help safeguard against kidney as well as urinary parcel contaminations. Ongoing investigations likewise show that cranberries assist with lessening awful cholesterol (LDL) and expands the degree of good cholesterol (HDL).

Ingredients:
- 1 cup berries, frozen
- 1 cup of water
- 1 tablespoon Splenda or 1 bundle Stevia
- 1 scoop vanilla whey seclude powder or 2 tablespoons gelatin in

addition to 1 teaspoon vanilla extract
- 2 teaspoon flaxseed oil
- 1 tablespoon ground flaxseed
- 1 teaspoon unsweetened cranberry juice
- 1 tablespoon lemon juice
- 10 ice cubes

Instructions:
1. Put each seemingly insignificant detail in a blender other than the ice.

Mix for until smooth. Incorporate the ice. Blend once more. Pour in a glass. Enjoy!

Serves: 2

Prep. Time: 4 minutes

Blend Time: 3 minutes

Dietetic Facts

Serving Size: 233 g

Calories: 193 Total

Fat: 8.5 g

Saturated Fat: 1 g Trans. Fat: 0 g

Cholesterol: 0 mg

Sodium: 34 mg

Potassium: 131 mg

Total Carbohydrates: 13.8 g Dietary Fiber: 3.4 g

Protein: 13.4 g

Vitamin A: 0%

Calcium: 3% Sugar: 9.2 g

Green and Blue Fruit Drink

henever I need to add greens into my Fruit Drink, spinach is my beloved green. It isn't quite so unpleasant as different greens, like kale, and they mix effectively to make scrumptious Fruit Drinks. Blueberries and spinach additionally consolidate to make a Fruit Drink that is loaded with Vitamin K, which is fundamental in bone wellbeing support, and too plentiful in vitamin A, folate, manganese, iron, and magnesium.

Ingredients:
- 1/3 cup frozen blueberries
- 1/4 cup unsweetened almond milk
- 1/2 cup Greek or Fage yogurt (plain or full-fat)
- 2 scoop vanilla seclude protein or 3 tablespoons gelatin in addition to 1

teaspoon vanilla extract
- 1 cup spinach, freely packed
- 1/4 cup ice

Instructions:
Put each easily overlooked detail in a blender other than the ice. Mix for

until smooth. Incorporate the ice. Blend once more. Include the ice blocks.

Mix once more. Pour in a glass. Enjoy!

Serves: 2

Prep. Time: 4 minutes

Blend Time: 3 minutes

Dietetic Facts

Serving Size: 384 g

Calories: 228 Total

Fat: 5 g

Saturated Fat: 3 g Trans. Fat: 0 g

Cholesterol: 7 mg

Sodium: 182 mg

Potassium: 445mg

Total Carbohydrates: 12.2 g Dietary

Fiber: 1.8 g

Protein: 37 g

Vitamin A: 58% Calcium: 28% Sugar: 8.9 g

Vitamin C: 24%

Iron: 11%

Blueberry Bliss

his basic low carb Fruit Drink is both nutritious and scrumptious. Beside
T

the sweet taste, blueberries are considered a superfood due to its high cell reinforcement content. Various examinations additionally show that blueberries help lower blood pressure and contain anti-diabetic effects. Like cranberries, blueberries also have anti-bacterial properties.

Ingredients:
- 1/4 cup frozen blueberries, unsweetened
- 1 bundle stevia or 1 tablespoon Splenda
- 1 scoop vanilla disengage protein or 2 tablespoons gelatin in addition to 1 teaspoon vanilla extract
- 15 ounces unsweetened almond milk, vanilla
- 5 ounces weighty cream

Instructions:
Put everything in a blender. Mix for until smooth. Pour in a glass. Enjoy!

Serves: 2
Prep. Time: 4 minutes
Blend Time: 3 minutes
Dietetic Facts
Serving Size: 322 g
Calories: 308 Total
Fat: 24.1 g
Saturated Fat: 14.3 g Trans. Fat: 0 g
Cholesterol: 77 mg
Sodium: 213 mg
Potassium: 234 mg
Total Carbohydrates: 10 g Dietary
Fiber: 1.4 g
Protein: 14.2 g Vitamin A: 18% Calcium: 35% Sugar: 5.6 g

Vitamin C: 6%
Iron: 5%

Berry Polka Dot Dance

his Fruit Drink will fulfill your sweet tooth with just 4.9 grams of net carbs. The flaxseeds pack the Fruit Drink with dietary fiber, micronutrients, vitamin B1, manganese, and heart-accommodating essential unsaturated fat omega 3 .

Ingredients:
- 1 cup unsweetened almond milk
- 1 cup spinach
- 2 tablespoons flax seeds
- 1/3 cup frozen blackberries
- 1/3 cup frozen blueberries
- 1 scoop vanilla detach protein or 2 tablespoons gelatin in addition to 1

teaspoon vanilla extract

Instructions:
1. Put everything in a blender. Mix for until smooth. Fill 2 glasses. Enjoy!

SERVES: 2
Prep. Time: 3 minutes
Blend Time: 2 minutes
Dietetic Facts
Serving Size: 268 g
Calories: 123 Total
Fat: 4 g
Saturated Fat: 0 g Trans. Fat: 0 g
Cholesterol: 0 mg
Sodium: 176 mg
Potassium: 314 mg
Total Carbohydrates: 8.8 g

Dietary Fiber: 3.9 g Sugar: 3.7 g
Protein: 14.3 g
Vitamin A: 29% Vitamin C: 22%

Spinach Avocado Banana Fruit Drink

T

his fast to make a heavenly Fruit Drink can be appreciated as a morning meal or bite drink. With a couple of fixings, this Fruit Drink is loaded with supplements that will give you the lift you really want in the morning. **Ingredients:**

- 2 cups spinach
- 1 enormous banana, frozen
- 1 avocado
- 1 tablespoon honey
- 1 pack gelatin or 1 scoop segregate protein
- 1 cup water
- 3 cups ice

Instructions:

Put all of the dynamic fixings into the blender or food processor.

Blend until smooth.

Serves: 5
Prep. Time: 3 minutes
Blend Time: 2 minutes
Dietetic Facts
Serving Size: 296 g
Calories: 197 Total
Fat: 8 g
Saturated Fat: 1.7 g Trans. Fat: 0 g
Cholesterol: 0 mg
Sodium: 62 mg
Potassium: 367 mg
Total Carbohydrates: 13.6 g Dietary
Fiber: 3.7 g Sugar: 7 g
Protein: 20.6 g
Vitamin A: 24% Vitamin C: 16%

Calcium: 4% **Iron:** 5%

Almond Avocado Fruit Drink

he key to this Fruit Drink is picking a decent almond spread. You will get the majority of your flavor from the almond margarine you pick. Almond spread contains copper and calcium, both of which play a vital role in keeping a solid sensory system and sound synapses. Almond spread is likewise plentiful in vitamin E, magnesium, fiber, and solid unsaturated fatty acids.

Ingredients:

- 1/2 avocado, stripped, pitted, sliced
- 1/2 cup half and half
- 1/2 cup unsweetened almond milk, vanilla
- 1/2 teaspoon vanilla extract
- 2 scoops vanilla detach protein
- 1 tablespoon almond butter
- Pinch of cinnamon
- 1 parcel stevia or 2 teaspoons Splenda
- 2-4 ice cubes

Instructions:

1. Put whatever in a blender other than the ice. Mix for until smooth. 2. Add in ice blocks. Mix again.

3. Pour in a glass. Enjoy!

Serves: 2

Prep. Time: 3 minutes

Blend Time: 2 minutes

Dietetic Facts

Serving Size: 214 g

Calories: 359 Total

Fat: 22.2 g

Saturated Fat: 6.9 g Trans. Fat: 0 g

Cholesterol: 22 mg

Sodium: 128 mg

Potassium: 437 mg

Total Carbohydrates: 13.1 g Dietary

Fiber: 4 g Sugar: 4.5 g

Protein: 28.7 g

Vitamin A: 6% **Vitamin C:** 9%

Almond Strawberry Glee

———————T

his reviving Fruit Drink is nutty with a smooth sweet taste. Beside antioxidants, strawberries also potassium, folate, dietary fiber, manganese. A portion of the medical advantages incorporate eye improvement and relief

cardiovascular-related diseases. **Ingredients:**
- 16 ounces unsweetened almond milk, vanilla
- 1 parcel stevia or 2 teaspoons Splenda
- 4 ounce weighty cream
- 2 scoops vanilla disengage protein or 4 tablespoons gelatin in addition

to 1 teaspoon vanilla extract
- 1/4 cup frozen strawberries, unsweetened

INSTRUCTIONS:
Put everything in a blender. Mix for until smooth. Pour in a glass.
Enjoy!
Serves: 2
Prep. Time: 3 minutes
Blend Time: 2 minutes
Dietetic Facts
Serving Size: 334 g
Calories: 352 Total
Fat: 24.2 g
Saturated Fat: 13.3 g Trans. Fat: 0 g
Cholesterol: 78 mg
Sodium: 240 mg
Potassium: 219 mg
Total Carbohydrates: 9 g
Dietary Fiber: 1.3 g Sugar: 5.2 g
Protein: 26 g

from arthritis, gout, high blood pressure, and various other

Creamy Blackberry

his beverage heavenly Fruit Drink is loaded with anthocyanin, which are
T

intensifies that assist with keeping the heart-sound. The fiber and magnesium of blackberries likewise advance solid blood stream and forestalls blockage in the

arteries, which reduces the risk of strokes and heart attacks.

Ingredients:

- 1 cup new blackberries
- 1 bundle stevia or 2 teaspoons Splenda
- 3/4 cup weighty whipping cream
- 2 scoops vanilla confine protein or 4 tablespoons gelatin in addition to 2

teaspoon vanilla extract

- 1 cup ice cubes

Instructions:

1. Placed whatever in a blender or food processor with the exception of

the ice. Blend for up until smooth.
2. Add in ice blocks. Mix again.
3. Pour in a glass. Enjoy!

Serves: 2
Prep. Time: 3 minutes
Blend Time: 2 minutes
Dietetic Facts
Serving Size: 268 g
Calories: 300 Total
Fat17 g
Saturated Fat: 10.4 g Trans. Fat: 0 g
Cholesterol:62 mg
Sodium: 76 mg
Potassium: 156 mg
Total Carbohydrates: 12.2 g
Dietary Fiber: 3.8 g Sugar: 7.6 g
Protein: 25.9 g

Spicy Green Salad Fruit Drink

hen you can't eat your plate of mixed greens, drink one! The primary

W

part of this Fruit Drink is white cabbage which is high in anthocyanins, and vitamin K Cabbage is additionally high in L-ascorbic acid, which detoxifies the body and

remove toxins.

Ingredients:

- 1 cup new white cabbage
- 1 modest bunch new child kale
- 1 modest bunch new parsley
- 1 lemon juice, fit into the blender
- 1 medium Roma or Heirloom tomato
- 1/2 cup water
- 1/2 habanero pepper, eliminate seeds
- 1/2 Italian cucumber
- 5-6 ice cubes

Optional:

- 1-2 tablespoon sunflower seeds
- Dash of cayenne pepper

Instructions:

4. Put everything in a blender with the exception of the ice 3D shapes.

Blend for until smooth.

5. Add in the ice 3D squares. Mix again.

6. Pour in a glass. Enjoy!

Serves: 2

Prep. Time: 3 minutes

Blend Time: 2 minutes

Dietetic Facts

Serving Size: 267 g

Calories: 51

Total Fat: 0.6 g

Saturated Fat: 0 g Trans. Fat: 0 g

Cholesterol: 0 mg

Sodium: 33 mg

Potassium: 470 mg

Total Carbohydrates: 10.4 g Dietary Fiber: 2.6 g

Protein: 2.6 g Vitamin A: 81% Calcium: 7% Sugar: 4.4 g

Vitamin C: 153%

Iron: 13%

Superfood Coconut Fruit Drink

I

f you love Coconut cream in your dessert, then you will love coconut cream in your Fruit Drink. Coconut cream, similar to coconut oil, is high antimicrobial mixtures, which successfully battles infections that cause measles, herpes, hepatitis, and the flu. The fats in coconut

cream are fat-consuming hydrogenated fat, which in itself is a characteristic enemy of oxidant that helps fight sans entirely free
 radicals. Moreover, coconut cream is cholesterol. Joined with blueberries, this Fruit Drink is really velvety and super healthy.

Ingredients:
- 1/2 cup coconut cream
- 1/2 cup frozen blueberries, unsweetened
- 1/2 cup unsweetened almond milk, vanilla
- 1 scoop vanilla disengage protein or 2 tablespoons gelatin in addition to 1 teaspoon vanilla extract
- 2-4 ice cubes

Instructions:
1. Put each seemingly insignificant detail in a blender other than the ice. Mix for until smooth.
2. Add in ice shapes. Mix again.
3. Pour in a glass. Enjoy!

Serves: 2
Prep. Time: 3 minutes
Blend Time: 2 minutes
Dietetic Facts
Serving Size: 173 g
Calories: 216 Total
Fat: 15.3 g
Saturated Fat: 12.8 g Trans. Fat: 0 g
Cholesterol: 0 mg
Sodium: 82 mg
Potassium: 235 mg
Total Carbohydrates: 9.1 g Dietary Fiber: 2.5 g
Protein: 13.9 g Vitamin A: 0% Calcium: 9% Sugar: 5.6 g

Vitamin C: 12%
Iron: 10%

Dairy-Free Green Fruit Drink

on't fret, the pineapple and the organic products in this Fruit Drink slice
D

directly through the greens. With the pineapple, this Fruit Drink can assist with restoring hacks, help weight reduction, reinforce bones, and lessen irritation. Pineapple is

also an excellent source of manganese and vitamin C.

Ingredients:
- 1 cup crude cucumber, stripped and sliced
- 1 cup romaine lettuce
- 1 tablespoon new ginger, stripped and chopped
- 1/2 cup kiwi organic product, stripped and chopped
- 1/2 Half avocado (eliminate pit and scoop the fully explore of shell)
- 1/3 cup hacked new pineapple
- 2 tablespoons new parsley
- 3 teaspoons Splenda
- 4 cups water

Instructions:
1. Put all of the fixings into the blender or food processor. Enjoy! **Serves:** 6
Prep Time: 5 minutes
Blend Time: 2 minutes
Dietetic Facts
Serving Size: 229 g
Calories: 63

Total Fat: 3.5 g
Saturated Fat: 0.7 g Trans. Fat: 0 g
Cholesterol: 0 mg
Sodium: 8 mg
Potassium: 196 mg
Total Carbohydrates: 8.4 g

Dietary Fiber: 2 g Sugar: 4.7 g
Protein: 0.8 g
Vitamin A: 3% Vitamin C: 37%
Calcium: 2% Iron: 4%

Coconut Chai Fruit Drink

T

his Fruit Drink is packed with anti-inflammatory, digestive, and cancer prevention agent properties. The almond spread adds wealth and a protein kick, while the flaxseeds add fiber and omega 3. Cinnamon decreases exhaustion, increment course, and increment essentialness. At last, ginger stimulates the invulnerable and circulatory system.

Ingredients:
- 1/4 cup unsweetened destroyed coconut
- 1 cup unsweetened coconut milk
- 1 tablespoon ground flaxseed
- 1 tablespoon unadulterated vanilla extract
- 1 teaspoon ground cinnamon
- 1 teaspoon ground ginger
- 2 tablespoons almond butter
- Pinch of allspice
- 5 ice cubes

Instructions:
1. Placed whatever in a blender or food processor aside from the ice shapes. Mix till its smooth.
2. Add in ice solid shapes. Mix again.
3. Pour in a glass. Enjoy!

SERVES: 2
Prep. Time: 3 minutes
Blend Time: 2 minutes
Dietetic Facts
Serving Size: 148 g
Calories: 421 Total
Fat: 38.8 g

Saturated Fat: 26.4 g Trans. Fat: 0 g Cholesterol: 0 mg
Sodium: 20 mg
Potassium: 493 mg
Total Carbohydrates: 13 g Dietary Fiber: 4.9 g
Protein: 6.9 g **Vitamin A:** 0% Calcium: 8% Sugar: 4.9 g

Vitamin C: 6%
Iron: 21%

Spicy Green Salad Fruit Drink

pice up your day with this fiery Fruit Drink. Assuming you like it hot,
S
you'll cherish this nutritious Fruit Drink that is loaded with nutrients and nutrients.

Ingredients:
- 1 cup new white cabbage
- 1 small bunch new child kale
- 1 small bunch new parsley
- 1 lemon juice, got into the blender
- 1 medium Roma or Heirloom tomato
- 1/2 cup water
- 1/2 habanero pepper, eliminate seeds
- 1/2 Italian cucumber
- 5-6 ice cubes

Optional:
- 1-2 tablespoon sunflower seeds
- Dash of cayenne pepper

1. Placed everything in a blender aside from the ice. Blend until its

smooth.
2. Add in the ice blocks. Mix again.
3. Pour in a glass. Enjoy!
Serves: 2
Prep. Time: 3 minutes
Blend Time: 2 minutes

DIETETIC FACTS

Serving Size: 267 g

Calories: 51

Total Fat: 0.6 g

Saturated Fat: 0 g Trans. Fat: 0 g

Cholesterol: 0 mg

Sodium: 33 mg

Potassium: 470 mg

Total Carbohydrates: 10.4 g Dietary Fiber: 2.6 g

Protein: 2.6 g Vitamin A: 81% Calcium: 7% Sugar: 4.4 g

Vitamin C: 153%

Iron: 13%

Orange Chocolate Fruit Drink

T

his Fruit Drink is a heavenly orange-chocolate charm. You will not figure that it's loaded with spinach. The orange concentrate additionally assists your body with engrossing the iron in spinach.

Ingredients:
- 1/8 teaspoon orange extract
- 1 cup unsweetened almond milk
- 1 scoop chocolate or vanilla seclude protein
- 1/2 cup spinach
- 2 tablespoons unsweetened cocoa powder

1. Put each easily overlooked detail in a blender other than the ice 3D

squares. Mix till its smooth.

2. Add in ice shapes. Mix again.

3. Pour in a glass. Enjoy!

Serves: 1

Prep. Time: 3 minutes

Blend Time: 2 minutes

Dietetic Facts

Serving Size: 304 g

Calories: 164 Total

Fat: 5.1 g

Saturated Fat: 1.2 g Trans. Fat: 0 g

Cholesterol: 0 mg

Sodium: 249 mg

Potassium: 444 mg

Total Carbohydrates: 8.5 g

Dietary Fiber: 4.9 g Sugar: 0 g

Protein: 27.5 g

Vitamin A: 28% Vitamin C: 7%

Calcium: 34% Iron: 16%

Green Minty Protein Shake

W

ho didn't adore chocolate chip frozen yogurt as a child? This delightful Fruit Drink will unquestionably fix your sweet tooth. It's so yummy, and you will not taste the greens. Incredible for youngsters too.

Ingredients:

- 1 parcel stevia or 2 teaspoons Splenda
- 1/4 teaspoon peppermint extract
- 1/2 cup almond milk, unsweetened
- 1/2 avocado
- 1 scoop vanilla or chocolate disengage protein
- 1 cup spinach, fresh
- 1 cup ice

Optional:

- Cacao nibs

Instructions:

1. Put each seemingly insignificant detail in a blender other than the ice blocks. Mix till its smooth.
2. Add in the ice 3D shapes. Mix again.
3. Pour in a glass. Enjoy!

Serves: 2

Prep Time: 3 minutes

Blend Time: 2 minutes

Dietetic Facts

Serving Size: 265 g

Calories: 184 Total

Fat: 10.8 g

Saturated Fat: 2.2 g Trans. Fat: 0 g

Cholesterol: 0 mg

Sodium: 91 mg

Potassium: 379 mg

Total Carbohydrates: 9.4 g Dietary

Fiber: 4 g

Protein: 13.6 g Vitamin A: 30% Calcium: 11% Sugar: 4.4 g

Vitamin C:15%

Iron: 6%

Peppermint Patty

T

his Fruit Drink has an aftertaste like a pepperMint patty yet is loaded with the nutritious integrity of spinach and almond milk. This drink is normally without sugar, Paleo-accommodating, sans gluten, sans dairy, and vegetarian. This Fruit Drink is thick and smooth with a frozen yogurt like goodness. Cocoa is wealthy in cholesterol-bringing down, disease battling cell reinforcement polyphenols. Mint, then again, is a characteristic catalyst and stomach related guide. You will adore the minty, chocolatey pleasantness of this Fruit Drink.

Ingredients:
- 1/4 teaspoon mint extract
- 1 scoop chocolate disengage protein
- 1 cup unsweetened almond milk
- 1 cup spinach
- 2 tbsp. unsweetened cocoa powder
- Ice cubes

Instructions:
1. Put each easily overlooked detail in a blender other than the ice solid

shapes. Mix till its smooth.

2. Add in ice solid shapes. Mix again.

3. Pour in a glass. Enjoy!

Serves: 1

Prep. Time: 3 minutes

Blend Time: 2 minutes

Dietetic Facts

Serving Size: 319 g

Calories: 166 Total

Fat: 5.1 g

Saturated Fat: 1.2 g Trans. Fat: 0 g

Cholesterol: 0 mg

Sodium: 261 mg

Potassium: 529 mg

Total Carbohydrates: 9 g Dietary Fiber: 5.3 g

Protein: 28 g

Vitamin A: 57% Calcium: 36% Sugar: 0 g

Vitamin C: 14%

Iron: 19%

Blue-Raspberry Fruit Drink

B

lueberries in addition to raspberries make this Fruit Drink a force to be reckoned with of antioxidants. Like blueberries,raspberries are rich in various cell reinforcements, like L-ascorbic acid, garlic corrosive, and quercetin, which help fight circulatory and heart diseases, cancer, and other age-related circumstances. Concentrates additionally show that entire eating berries are more beneficial than taking them in dietary enhancement form.

Ingredients:
- 1/4 cup blueberries, frozen

- 1/4 cup raspberries, frozen
- 1 1/2 cups unsweetened almond milk
- 1 pack gelatin or 1 scoop segregate protein

INSTRUCTIONS:
Put all of the fixings into the blender or food processor. Mix until smooth. **Serves:** 1
Prep. Time: 3 minutes
Blend Time: 2 minutes
Dietetic Facts
Serving Size: 470 g
Calories: 191 Total
Fat: 5.6g
Saturated Fat: 0 g Trans. Fat: 0 g
Cholesterol: 0 mg
Sodium: 325 mg
Potassium: 364 mg
Total Carbohydrates: 11.9 g
Dietary Fiber: 4.4 g Sugar: 5 g

Protein: 26.1 g
Vitamin A: 0% Vitamin C: 23%
Calcium: 47% Iron: 12%

Kale, Spinach, and Strawberry Fruit Drink

Kbeer is a superfood that is loaded with nutrients K, C, and A. The mix of Kale and Spinach makes this Fruit Drink a super punch of nutrients!. **Ingredients:**
- 2 cups kale
- 1 cup spinach
- 1/4 cup strawberries

- 1 cup unsweetened almond milk
- 2 packs gelatin

Instructions:

1. Put all of the fixings into the blender or food processor. Mix until smooth.

Serves: 2

Prep. Time: 3 minutes

Blend Time: 2 minutes

Dietetic Facts

Serving Size: 253 g

Calories: 156 Total

Fat: 1.9 g

Saturated Fat: 0 g Trans. Fat: 0 g

Cholesterol: 0 mg

Sodium: 186 mg

Potassium: 540 mg

Total Carbohydrates: 9.9 g

Dietary Fiber: 2.2 g Sugar: 0.9 g

Protein: 27 g

Vitamin A: 234% Vitamin C: 159%

Calcium: 27% Iron: 12%

Green Power Fruit Drink

T

his Fruit Drink is packed whole food goodness of kale, spinach, blueberries, strawberries, ginger, egg, and flax seeds. But what really makes this recipe is the creamy texture of yogurt. Greek yogurt is loaded with probiotics that assist with keeping a good overall arrangement of good microscopic organisms in your stomach related framework. It's likewise loaded with vitamin B12 that helps maintain solid cerebrum function.

Ingredients:

- 12 ounce Greek yogurt
- 1 cup spinach
- 1 cup kale
- 1/2 cup strawberry
- 1/2 cup blueberries
- 1 cup of water
- 2 tbsp. flax seeds
- 1 tsp. ginger root, grated
- 1 egg
- 4 pack gelatin or 4 scoops segregate protein
- 1 ounce lemon zest

Instructions:

1. Put all of the fixings into the blender or food processor. Mix until

smooth.

Serves: 4

Prep. Time: 3 minutes

Blend Time: 2 minutes

Dietetic Facts

Serving Size: 255 g

Calories: 221 Total

Fat: 4.1 g

Saturated Fat: 1.8 g Trans. Fat: 0 g

Cholesterol: 45 mg

Sodium: 115 mg

Potassium: 345 mg

Total Carbohydrates: 11.3 g Dietary Fiber:

2.4 g Sugar: 6.5 g

Protein: 35.6 g

Vitamin A: 67% Vitamin C: 66%

Calcium: 14% Iron: 13%

Red Heart Fruit Drink

———◈——— T

his red Fruit Drink is stuffed flavonoids from the red cabbages, which likewise gives its red tone. The red cabbage is loaded with L-ascorbic acid, and 1 cup contains 56% of your body's every day suggested admission. Red cabbage likewise wraps this Fruit Drink with phytochemicals that help reduce the danger of coronary illness, disease, and other

illnesses.

Ingredients:
- 5 medium strawberries
- 1/2 cup raspberries
- 1 cup red cabbage, chopped
- 1/2 red chime pepper
- 1 roma tomato
- 8 oz. cold water
- 1 ice cube

Instructions:

1. Put all of the fixings into the blender or food processor. Mix until

smooth.

Serves: 2

Prep. Time: 3 minutes

Blend Time: 2 minutes

Dietetic Facts

Serving Size: 360 g

Calories: 1157

Total Fat: 0.7 g

Saturated Fat: 0 g Trans. Fat: 0 g

Cholesterol: 0 mg

Sodium: 74 mg

Potassium: 2425 mg

Total Carbohydrates: 14.3 g

Dietary Fiber: 5.1 g Sugar: 7.7 g

Protein: 26.3 g
Vitamin A: 20% Vitamin C: 178%
Calcium: 5% **Iron:** 16%

Orange-Carrot Fruit Drink

his Fruit Drink is loaded with the integrity of carrots yet suggests a flavor
T

like oranges. Carrots load this beverage with beta-carotene or vitamin A. They are wealthy in fiber and are a decent wellspring of nutrients K, C, B8, folate,

pantothenic acid, iron, potassium, manganese, and copper.

Ingredients:
- 1 cup cut carrots
- 3/4 cup orange juice
- 1/2 teaspoon orange peel
- 3 pack gelatin or 3 scoops disengage protein
- 1 1/2 cups ice cubes

Instructions:
1. Put all of the fixings into the blender or food processor. Mix until

smooth.

Serves: 3
Prep. Time: 3 minutes
Blend Time: 2 minutes
Dietetic Facts
Serving Size: 246 g
Calories: 137 Total
Fat: 0.2 g
Saturated Fat: 0 g Trans. Fat: 0 g
Cholesterol: 0 mg
Sodium: 84 mg
Potassium: 248 mg
Total Carbohydrates: 10.1 g Dietary
Fiber: 1.1 g Sugar: 7 g
Protein: 24.7 g
Vitamin A: 123% Vitamin C: 91%
Calcium: 3% **Iron:** 7%

Super Green Fruit Drink

I n this formula, we make a special case for oats and just add a little to add

to the thickness of the Fruit Drink. Oats are wealthy in solvent fiber that exploration shows they might assist with diminishing the danger of coronary illness, colorectal *cancer, and blood pressure.*

Ingredients:

- 6 ounces unsweetened almond milk
- 3 tablespoon rolled oats
- 1 cup spinach
- 2 strawberries
- 1/2 cup blueberries
- 1/2 stem celery
- 3 cuts cucumber
- 1 teaspoon cinnamon
- 1 tablespoon flax seed
- 1 tablespoon cocoa powder
- 4 pack gelatin

Instructions:

1. Put all of the fixings into the blender or food processor. Mix until

smooth.

Serves: 5

Prep. Time: 3 minutes

Blend Time: 2 minutes

Dietetic Facts

Serving Size: 267 g

Calories: 141 Total

Fat: 1.6 g

Saturated Fat: 0 g Trans. Fat: 0 g

Cholesterol: 0 mg

Sodium: 77 mg

Potassium: 376 mg

Total Carbohydrates: 12.9 g Dietary Fiber:

2.9 g Sugar: 4.8 g

Protein: 21.6 g

Vitamin A: 10% Vitamin C: 18%

Calcium: 9% **Iron:** 10%

Superfood Fruit Drink

———S

pinach is a notable superfood at this point that is loaded with astounding medical advantages, which incorporate further developing the blood glucose control and bone wellbeing, bringing down the danger of asthma and pulse. Spinach likewise contains alpha-lipoic corrosive or ALA, which assists with lessening glucose level and increment insulin

sensitivity.

Ingredients:

- 100 g Greek yogurt
- 1/2 avocado
- 1/3 cup strawberries, frozen
- 1/2 cup blueberries, frozen
- 3/4 cup unsweetened almond milk
- 2 tablespoons flaxseed
- 1 cup spinach
- 2 packs gelatin

Instructions:

1. Put all of the fixings into the blender or food processor. Mix until smooth.
  Serves: 2
  Prep. Time: 3 minutes
  Blend Time: 2 minutes
  Nutritional Facts
  Serving Size: 304 g
  Calories: 318
  Total Fat: 14.6 g
  Saturated Fat: 3.3 g Trans. Fat: 0 g
  Cholesterol: 3 mg
  Sodium: 156 mg
  Potassium: 595 mg
  Total Carbohydrates: 16.7 g
  Dietary Fiber: 7.3 g Sugar: 7.2 g
  Protein: 32.5 g
  Vitamin A: 30% Vitamin C: 49%
  Calcium: 21% Iron: 22%

Silken Tofu Fruit Drink

S

trawberries, tofu, and almond organization to make a basic yet exceptionally fulfilling velvety Fruit Drink that is normally high in protein. Makes for an incredible post-exercise Fruit Drink!

Ingredients:
- 1/2 cup strawberries, unfrozen
- 1 cut smooth tofu
- 1 cup unsweetened almond milk, vanilla
- Pinch of cinnamon
- 1 bundle stevia or 2 teaspoons Splenda

Instructions:
2. Put everything in a blender. Mix for until smooth. Pour in a glass.

Enjoy!

Serves: 2

Prep. Time: 3 minutes

Blend Time: 2 minutes

Dietetic Facts

Serving Size: 225 g

Calories: 145 Total

Fat: 3.0 g

Saturated Fat: 0 g Trans. Fat: 0 g

Cholesterol: 0 mg

Sodium: 133 mg

Potassium: 234 mg

Total Carbohydrates: 12.9 g Dietary

Fiber: 1.3 g

Protein: 15.6 g Vitamin A: 0% Calcium: 18% Sugar: 10.3 g

Vitamin C: 35%

Iron: 6%

Carrot and Leafy Green Fruit Drink

uper greens, carrots, and peaches make this an invigorating Fruit Drink

S

that is loaded with vitamin An and cancer prevention agents. Amazing on a warm summer day!

Ingredients:

- 1/2 cup peach cuts, frozen
- 1 medium carrot
- 1/2 cup green grapes
- 1/2 cup spinach
- 1/2 cup green cabbage
- 1/2 cup unsweetened almond milk
- 1 tablespoon ground flaxseeds
- 1/2 cup ice cubes
- 2 pack gelatin

Instructions:

1. Put all of the fixings into the blender or food processor. Mix until smooth.

Serves: 2

Net Carb: 10.4 g Prep.

Time: 3 minutes Blend

Time: 2 minutes

Dietetic Facts

Serving Size: 274g

Calories: 173

Total Fat: 2.2 g

Saturated Fat: 0 g Trans. Fat: 0 g

Cholesterol: 0 mg

Sodium: 133 mg

Potassium: 375 mg

Total Carbohydrates: 13.8 g

Dietary Fiber: 3.4 g Sugar: 9.4 g

Protein: 26.1 g

Vitamin A: 120% Vitamin C: 23%

Calcium: 12% Iron: 11%

Mango-Carrot Green Tea Fruit Drinks

T

his Fruit Drink requires a touch of exertion, yet everything will work out. Green tea sets with different flavors well. The blend of carrots, mango, and ginger makes for an extraordinary tasting Fruit Drink. **Ingredients:**

- 5 ounces mango, frozen
- 1 cup carrots
- 1-inch tablespoon ginger pounded
- 4 green tea bags
- 1 teaspoon honey
- 1 tablespoon chia seeds or flax seeds
- 4 pack gelatin
- 3 cups water

Instructions:

1. In a little pot, pour water. Heat water to the point of boiling. Include

the carrots. Cover. Cook for around 10-15 mins or until the carrots hurt. Include the ginger during the most recent 2 minutes of cooking.

2. Remove the pot from the hotness. Include the tea sacks. Cover. Steep for 4 minutes. Eliminate the tea sacks, crushing out all the tea. Dispose of the ginger. Keep the container on a hot cushion in the ice chest for 10 minutes.

3. Transfer the carrot combination into a blender. Include the mango. Add in the chia or flax seeds.

4. Blend until smooth. Serve.

Serves: 4

Prep. Time: 35 minutes

Blend Time: 2 minutes

Dietetic Facts

Serving Size: 276

g Calories: 149

Total Fat: 0.8 g

Saturated Fat: 0 g Trans. Fat: 0 g

Cholesterol: 0 mg

Sodium: 81 mg

Potassium: 198 mg

Total Carbohydrates: 11.6 g Dietary

Fiber: 2 g Sugar: 8.2 g

Protein: 24.8 g

Vitamin A: 970% Vitamin C: 19%

Calcium: 4% Iron: 6%

Part Two:

Charming Fruit Drinks

hese Fruit Drinks are keto-accommodating treats in a cup! You can have these delightful beverages without stressing over having an excessive number of carbs. Simply remember what your objective marco's are for the afternoon and appreciate it!

Creamy Chocolate Milkshake

———T

his is an extremely simple as well as fast means to make your own keto wonderful, scrumptious chocolate milkshake or smoothie. This low carb rendition is scrumptious, but since you can eat a great deal of fat, you can appreciate it irreproachable! Ingredients:

- 16 ounces unsweetened almond milk, vanilla
- 4 ounces weighty cream
- 1 scoop chocolate detach protein
- 1 bundle stevia or 2 teaspoons Splenda
- 1/2 cup squashed ice

Instructions:

1. Put each easily overlooked detail in a blender or food processor with

the exception of the ice. Mix for until smooth.

2. Add in the ice shapes. Mix again.

3. Pour in a glass. Enjoy!

Serves: 2

Prep. Time: 3 minutes

Blend Time: 2 minutes

Dietetic Facts

Serving Size: 361 g

Calories: 120 Total

Fat: 24.2 g

Saturated Fat: 13.3 g Trans. Fat: 0 g

Cholesterol: 78 mg

Sodium: 214 mg

Potassium: 218 mg

Total Carbohydrates: 7.4 g

Dietary Fiber: 0.9 g Sugar: 4.1 g

Protein: 14.1 g

Vitamin A: 17% Vitamin C: 1%

Calcium: 32% Iron: 5%

Espresso Fruit Drink

Y

ou 'll adore the smell and intense, severe kind of this beverage. Espresso keeps you alert, yet there is research that shows drinking a cup of Joe builds insulin responsiveness because of its mineral substance of chromium and magnesium., These are known to animate insulin take-up in the cells. Espresso is likewise an extraordinary wellspring of cancer prevention agents, which are known to bring down chances of incendiary circumstances, for example, Alzheimer's and Parkinson's disease. **Ingredients:**

- 1/4 cup (65 g) Greek yogurt, full-fat
- 1 coffee shot or 1 mug dark coffee
- 1 scoop vanilla separate protein or 2 tablespoons gelatin in addition to 1 teaspoon vanilla extract
- 1/2 parcel stevia or 1 teaspoon Splenda
- Pinch of cinnamon
- 5 ice cubes

Instructions:

- Put each easily overlooked detail in a blender or food processor aside from the ice. Mix for until smooth.
- Add in the ice solid shapes. Mix again.
- Pour in a glass. Enjoy!

Serves: 1

Prep. Time: 3 minutes

Blend Time: 2 minutes

Dietetic Facts

Serving Size: 338

g Calories: 186

Total Fat: 1.4 g

Saturated Fat: 1.0 g Trans. Fat: 0 g

Cholesterol: 3 mg

Sodium: 81 mg

Potassium: 214 mg

Total Carbohydrates: 10.9 g Dietary Fiber:

0 g

Protein: 30.8 g **Vitamin A:** 0% Calcium: 9% Sugar: 10.6 g

Vitamin C: 0%

Iron: 2%

Hazelnut Keto Coffee Fruit Drink

——————T

his Fruit Drink joins hazelnut flavor and espresso into a delectable sweet that will get your day going with a scrumptious bang!

Ingredients:
- 1/3 cup weighty cream
- 1 mug cold coffee
- 1-2 tablespoon hazelnut syrup, sugar-free
- Ice cubes

Instructions:

1. Put each seemingly insignificant detail in a blender or food processor

aside from the ice. Mix for until smooth.

2. Add in ice 3D squares. Mix again.

3. Pour in a glass. Enjoy!

Serves: 1

Prep. Time: 3 minutes

Blend Time: 2 minutes

Dietetic Facts

Serving Size: 286 g

Calories: 19

Total Fat: 20.6 g

Saturated Fat: 9.6 g Trans. Fat: 0 g

Cholesterol: 55 mg

Sodium: 20 mg

Potassium: 210 mg

Total Carbohydrates: 2.7 g

Dietary Fiber: 0.9 g Sugar: 0 g

Protein: 2.5 g

The Peanut Milkshake

eanut spread isn't only for your child's lunch! This adaptable spread is

P

high in sound oils and protein, which assist with helping weight reduction, diabetes, and Alzheimer's illness. Peanuts likewise contain fiber for a sound bowel

movement, magnesium for muscle and bone health.

Ingredients:

• 2 tablespoons peanut butter, all-natural

• 1 tsp vanilla extract

• 1 parcel stevia or 2 teaspoons Splenda

• 1 cup unsweetened almond milk, vanilla

• 1/2 cup coconut milk, regular

• 1 cup of ice cubes

Instructions:

1. Put each easily overlooked detail in a blender or food processor with

the exception of the ice. Mix for until smooth.

2. Add in ice 3D squares. Mix again.

3. Pour in a glass. Enjoy!

Serves: 2

Prep. Time: 3 minutes

Blend Time: 2 minutes

Dietetic Facts

Serving Size: 326g

Calories: 278

Total Fat: 24.1 g

Saturated Fat: 14.5 g Trans. Fat: 0 g

Cholesterol: 0 mg

Sodium: 176 mg

Potassium: 361 mg

Total Carbohydrates: 11.7g

Dietary Fiber: 2.8 g Sugar: 7.8 g

Protein: 5.9 g

The Keto Frapp

his without dairy, without sugar, totally keto, and vegetarian agreeable
T

Fruit Drink is an extraordinary method consuming morning. This straightforward sneaks added supplements in with grounded flax seeds.

Ingredients:

- 1 cup extra or cold coffee
- 1 teaspoon vanilla extract
- 1/3 cup weighty cream
- 1-2 tablespoons ground flax seeds
- 6 ice cubes

Optional: for a sweeter blend

- 2 tablespoons salted caramel syrup, sugar-free

Instructions:

1. Put each seemingly insignificant detail in a blender or food processor

aside from the ice. Mix for until smooth.

2. Add in ice 3D squares. Mix again.

3. Pour in a glass.

4. Add caramel syrup, whenever wanted. Enjoy!

Serves: 1

Prep. Time: 3 minutes

Blend Time: 2 minutes

Dietetic Facts

Serving Size: 295 g

Calories: 226 Total

Fat: 19.5 g

Saturated Fat: 9.8 g Trans. Fat: 0 g

Cholesterol: 55 mg

Sodium: 24 mg

Potassium: 266 mg

Total Carbohydrates: 5.7 g Dietary: 0g

Fiber: 3.8 g Sugar: 0.8 g

Protein: 3.7 g

Vitamin A: 12% Vitamin C: 0%

for starting off your fatand scrumptious beverage Calcium: 4% Iron: 22%

Apricot, Peach, and Coconut Fruit Drink

A

pricots mix well with coconut and other tropical natural products. Mixing them with peaches and coconut milk is a yummy alternative.

Ingredients:

· 6 ounces coconut milk

· 1 cup peaches

· 1 1/2 cup apricot

· 4 pack gelatin

· 1 cup ice 3D shapes

Instructions:

1. Place each of the dynamic fixings solidly into the blender. Mix until

smooth.

Serves: 4
Prep. Time: 3 minutes
Blend Time: 2 minutes
Dietetic Facts
Serving Size: 230g
Calories: 236
Total Fat: 10.6 g
Saturated Fat: 9 g Trans. Fat: 0 g
Cholesterol: 0 mg
Sodium: 64 mg
Potassium: 348 mg
Total Carbohydrates: 12.8 g
Dietary Fiber: 2.7 g Sugar: 10.2 g
Protein: 26.1 g
Vitamin A: 25% Vitamin C: 16%
Calcium: 3% **Iron:** 7%

Rich n' Creamy Blackberry Fruit Drink

lackberries make this Fruit Drink plentiful in Vitamin C and bioflavonoids. These berries have one of the greatest antioxidant degrees of all fruits, which provide their dark blue shade. Bioflavonoids assist with making the skin look more youthful, keeps the cerebrum alarm, and keeps up with your memory. Blueberries are likewise high in tannin, which helps you 'down there' by assisting with mitigating hemorrhoids, lessen irritation in the digestive tract, and soothe diarrhea.

Ingredients:
- 1 cup new blackberries
- 1 bundle stevia or 2 teaspoons Splenda
- 3/4 cup weighty whipping cream
- 2 scoops vanilla disconnect protein or 4 tablespoons gelatin in addition

to 2 teaspoon vanilla extract
• 1 cup ice cubes
Instructions:
1. Put each easily overlooked detail in a blender or food processor aside

from the ice. Mix for until smooth.
2. Add in ice 3D shapes. Mix again.
3. Pour in a glass. Enjoy!
Serves: 2
Prep. Time: 3 minutes
Blend Time: 2 minutes
Dietetic Facts
Serving Size: 268
g Calories: 300
Total Fat17 g
Saturated Fat: 10.4 g Trans. Fat: 0 g
Cholesterol: 62 mg
Sodium: 76 mg
Potassium: 156 mg
Total Carbohydrates: 12.2 g Dietary
Fiber: 3.8 g Sugar: 7.6 g
Protein: 25.9 g
Vitamin A: 16% Vitamin C: 26%
Calcium: 7% Iron: 4%

Cinnamon Roll Fruit Drink

———————T

his tasty Fruit Drink contains Chia seeds, which are loaded with supplements. Indeed, chia is an antiquated Mayan word for "strength". These seeds are stacked with protein, fiber, omega 3 unsaturated fats, and different micronutrients. They are additionally wealthy in calcium, magnesium, manganese, and phosphorus.

Ingredients:

- 1/4 tsp vanilla extract
- 1/2 tsp cinnamon
- 1 cup unsweetened almond milk
- 1 bundle stevia
- 1 tbsp. chia seeds or flax seeds
- 2 tbsp. vanilla protein powder or 2 tablespoons gelatin in addition to 1

teaspoon vanilla extract
- 1 cup ice cubes

Instructions:

1. Put each easily overlooked detail in a blender or food processor aside

from the ice. Mix until smooth.

2. Add in the ice solid shapes. Mix again.

3. Pour in a glass. Enjoy!

Serves: 1

Prep. Time: 3 minutes

Blend Time: 2 minutes

Dietetic Facts

Serving Size: 532 g

Calories: 217 Total

Fat: 24.2 g

Saturated Fat: 0.6 g Trans. Fat: 0 g

Cholesterol: 0 mg

Sodium: 244 mg

Potassium: 260 mg

Total Carbohydrates: 13.1 g Dietary

Fiber: 3.5 g Sugar: 8.2 g

Protein: 26.3 g **Vitamin A:** 0% Calcium: 34%

Vitamin C: 0%

Iron: 17%

Yummy Strawberry-Cheesecake Fruit Drink

———⊗⊗⊗——— T

his basic velvety thick Fruit Drink is sweet and has a liberal strawberry cheesecake flavor that will fulfill your taste buds. The mystery of this drink is the integrity of cream cheddar, which gives it that creamy

tangy taste that we all love.

Ingredients:

- 1/2 cup frozen strawberries, unsweetened
- 1/2 cup unsweetened almond milk, vanilla
- 1/2 teaspoons vanilla extract
- 2 ounces cream cheddar, regular
- 2 parcels stevia or 4 teaspoons Splenda
- 3-4 ice cubes

Instructions:

1. Put each seemingly insignificant detail in a blender or food processor

with the exception of the ice. Mix until smooth.

2. Add in ice solid shapes. Mix again.
3. Pour in a glass. Enjoy!

Serves: 2

Prep. Time: 3 minutes

Blend Time: 2 minutes

Dietetic Facts

Serving Size: 138

g Calories: 164

Total Fat: 10.8 g

Saturated Fat: 6.3 g Trans. Fat: 0 g

Cholesterol: 31 mg

Sodium: 129 mg

Potassium: 83 mg

Total Carbohydrates: 12.6 g

Dietary Fiber: 1 g Protein: 2.4 g

Vitamin A: 8% Calcium: 10% Sugar: 10.4 g

Mango Berry Slush

T *his mix is a scrumptiously tart and sweet beverage that is loaded with*

vitamin

C. *This berry flavored slushy is a refreshing low-carb, high protein drink that everyone will love.*

Ingredients:
- 4 ounces' mango
- 1 cup strawberries
- 1 1/2 cups carbonated water
- 1 1/2 cups ice
- 4 pack gelatin
- 1 lime

Instructions:
1. Put all of the parts solidly into the blender or food processor. Mix until smooth.

Serves: 4
Prep. Time: 3 minutes
Blend Time: 2 minutes
Dietetic Facts
Serving Size: 281 g
Calories: 128 Total
Fat: 0.2 g
Saturated Fat: 0 g Trans. Fat: 0 g
Cholesterol: 0 mg
Sodium: 60 mg
Potassium: 117 mg
Total Carbohydrates: 8.5 g
Dietary Fiber: 1.3 g Sugar: 6.2 g
Protein: 24.4 g
Vitamin A: 5% Vitamin C: 54%

Raspberry Cheesecake Blend

L

ike the Strawberry-Cheesecake Fruit Drink, this variant is a yummy Fruit Drink with a rich, sweet cheesecake flavor. The curds includes protein with everything else and keeps the carbs low. The protein content of this

cheese is casein, which make you feel full longer and helps build muscle. **Ingredients:**
- 1 cup unsweetened almond milk
- 1/2 cup raspberries
- 1 ounce cream cheese
- 1 tablespoon vanilla syrup, sugar-free
- 4 Ice cubes

Instructions:

1. Put each seemingly insignificant detail in a blender or food processor

with the exception of the ice. Mix for until smooth.

2. Add in ice 3D shapes. Mix again.

3. Pour in a glass. Enjoy!

Serves: 1

Prep. Time: 3 minutes

Blend Time: 2 minutes

Dietetic Facts

Serving Size: 353 g

Calories: 208 Total

Fat: 13.8 g

Saturated Fat: 6.5 g Trans. Fat: 0 g

Cholesterol: 31 mg

Sodium: 266 mg

Potassium: 336 mg

Total Carbohydrates: 11.7 g Dietary

Fiber: 5.0 g Sugar: 4.4 g

Protein: 3.9 g

Vitamin A: 8% Vitamin C: 27%

Calcium: 34% Iron: 8%

Strawberry-Almond Crunch Fruit Drink

A *dding almond nuts to a strawberry Fruit Drink gives it a tasty crunchy*

surface. It additionally packs the Fruit Drink the supplements L-carnitine (known for its weight reduction properties) and riboflavin, which help boost

brain activity and reduce the risk of Alzhei mer's disease.

Ingredients:

- 2 tablespoons almonds
- 1/2 teaspoon cinnamon
- 1/2 cup natural strawberries, frozen
- 1 cup unsweetened almond milk, vanilla
- 2 chilled cubes

OPTIONAL:
• 1 tablespoon chia seeds or flax seeds
Instructions:
1. Put everything in a blender. Mix for until smooth. Pour in a glass. Add

chilled shapes and enjoy!
Serves: 1
Prep. Time: 3 minutes
Blend Time: 2 minutes
Dietetic Facts
Serving Size: 335 g
Calories: 135 Total
Fat: 9.7 g
Saturated Fat: 0.8 g Trans. Fat: 0 g
Cholesterol: 0 mg
Sodium: 181 mg
Potassium: 392 mg
Total Carbohydrates: 11 g

Dietary Fiber: 4.5 g Sugar: 4 g
Protein: 4 g
Vitamin A: 0% Calcium: 36% Vitamin C: 71%

Iron: 9%

Peach Pie Shake

T his sweet-smelling Fruit Drink is sweet and tart. Peach is a decent

wellspring of vitamin A that further develops vision and assists battle with liberating extremists. Nutrients An and C keeps skin sound - saturated, sparkling, graceful, and soft.

Regularly eating peaches also helps increase the blood circulation of the body.

Ingredients:

• 1 peach, pitted

• 1 scoop vanilla protein powder or 2 tablespoons gelatin in addition to 1 teaspoon vanilla extract

• 1/4 cup plain Greek yogurt

• 2 portions of cinnamon

• 2/3 cup unsweetened almond milk

• 8-10 ice cubes

Instructions:

• Put each easily overlooked detail in a blender or food processor aside from the ice. Mix for until smooth.

• Add in the ice blocks. Mix again.

• Pour in a glass. Enjoy!

Serves: 1

Prep. Time: 3 minutes

Blend Time: 2 minutes

Dietetic Facts

Serving Size: 358 g

Calories: 209 Total

Fat: 3.9 g

Saturated Fat: 1.2 g Trans. Fat: 0 g

Cholesterol: 3 mg

Sodium: 196 mg

Potassium: 412 mg

Total Carbohydrates: 13.8 g Dietary Fiber: 2.5 g

Protein: 32.1 g Vitamin A: 7% Calcium: 29% Sugar: 10.8 g

Vitamin C: 11%

Iron: 6%

Buttered Pumpkin Pie Coffee

W*hile the vast majority of the pumpkin-seasoned treats ought to be* *appreciated infrequently, you can taste on this low carb natural product drink consistently. Besides, this faultless Fruit Drink is loaded with 102% of your day by day admission of nutrient A.*

Ingredients:
- 1/4 teaspoon pumpkin pie spice
- 1 tablespoon ordinary margarine, unsalted
- 12 ounces hot coffee
- 2 tablespoons canned pumpkin
- 1 bundle stevia or 2 teaspoons Splenda

Instructions:
- Put everything in a blender. Mix for until smooth. Pour in a glass.

Enjoy!

Serves: 1

Prep. Time: 3 minutes

Blend Time: 2 minutes

Dietetic Facts

Serving Size: 393 g

Calories: 157 Total

Fat: 11.7 g

Saturated Fat: 7.4 g Trans. Fat: 0 g

Cholesterol: 31 mg

Sodium: 90 mg

Potassium: 236 mg

Total Carbohydrates: 10.8 g Dietary

Fiber: 0.9 g Sugar: 9.1 g

Protein: 0.9 g

Vitamin A: 102% Vitamin C: 2%

Calcium: 2% Iron: 3%

Chocolate-Cayenne Shake

his Fruit Drink is an exceptional treat. This chilly mix is spiked with the
T

astonishing hint of cayenne heat. Cayenne is a zest known to kill sharpness and invigorate course. This spreads the word about it a well ingredient

in detoxifying and cleansing regimes.

Ingredients:

- 1/4 cup coconut cream
- 1/2 - 1 cup water
- 1/2 squeeze cayenne powder
- 1 tbsp. flax seeds or chia seeds
- 2 tbsp. unsweetened cocoa powder
- 2 tbsp. raw coconut oil
- Dash of vanilla extract
- Pinch of ground cinnamon
- Ice shapes, if desired

Instructions:

1. Put each seemingly insignificant detail in a blender or food processor aside from the ice. Mix for until smooth.
2. Add in the ice 3D squares. Mix again.
3. Pour in a glass. Enjoy!

Serves: 2

Prep. Time: 3 minutes

Blend Time: 2 minutes

Dietetic Facts

Serving Size: 171 g

Calories: 218 Total

Fat: 22.6 g

Saturated Fat: 18.7 g Trans. Fat: 0 g

Cholesterol: 0 mg

Sodium: 10 mg

Potassium: 246 mg

Total Carbohydrates: 5.8 g Dietary Fiber:

3.3 g Sugar: 1.2 g

Protein: 2.3 g **Vitamin A:** 1% Calcium: 2%

Vitamin C: 2%

Iron: 13%

Peanut Butter Crunch Chocolate Fruit Drink

T

his smooth thick Fruit Drink is a nutritious breakfast or as a liberal tidbit. This Fruit Drink will fuel you and fulfill your sweet tooth.

Ingredients:
- 1 1/2 cups unsweetened almond milk
- 1 1/2scoop chocolate whey protein powder 2 tablespoons gelatin in

addition to 11/2 tablespoon unsweetened cocoa powder
- 1 bundle stevia or 2 teaspoons Splenda
- 2 tablespoons peanut butter, organic
- 1/2 cup ice

Instructions:
1. Put everything in a blender. Mix for until smooth. Change pleasantness

as per taste.
2. Pour in a glass. Enjoy!

Serves: 2
Prep. Time: 3 minutes
Blend Time: 2 minutes
Dietetic Facts
Serving Size: 338 g
Calories: 186 Total
Fat: 1.4 g
Saturated Fat: 1 g Trans. Fat: 0 g
Cholesterol: 3 mg
Sodium: 81 mg
Potassium: 214 mg
Total Carbohydrates: 10.9 g Dietary
Fiber: 0 g Sugar: 10.6 g
Protein: 30.8 g
Vitamin A: 0% **Vitamin C:** 0%

Calcium: 9% Iron: 2%

Whipped Chocolate Shake

————W

hipping cream makes this shake light as air and smooth. This off the charts shocking beverage is likewise high in calcium.

Ingredients:
- 1 cup unsweetened almond milk
- 1/3 cup weighty whipping cream
- 1 parcel stevia or 2 teaspoons Splenda
- 1/2 teaspoon vanilla extract
- 1 tablespoon unsweetened cocoa powder
- 3 ice cubes

Instructions:
1. Put each easily overlooked detail in a blender or food processor aside

from the ice. Mix for until smooth.
2. Add in ice 3D shapes. Mix again.
3. Pour in a glass. Enjoy!

Serves: 1
Prep. Time: 3 minutes
Blend Time: 2 minutes
Dietetic Facts
Serving Size: 306 g
Calories: 236 Total
Fat: 19 g
Saturated Fat: 10 g Trans. Fat: 0 g
Cholesterol: 55 mg
Sodium: 197 mg
Potassium: 305 mg
Total Carbohydrates: 14.3 g Dietary
Fiber: 2.8 g Sugar: 8.4g
Protein: 2.9 g

Mango Almond Fruit Drink

Here's a straightforward, simple, sound, yet heavenly vegetarian and low

fat Fruit Drink. Research shows that Mangoes are loaded with cell reinforcements that help safeguard against leukemia, bosom, colon, and prostate malignant growth. Mangoes

are also high in pectin, fiber, and vitamin C that lower LDL or bad cholesterol. They also help keep the skin clear, improve eye health, improve digestion, and boost the immune system.

Ingredients:
- 125 g mango, frozen
- 3/4 cup unsweetened almond milk
- 1 pack gelatin or 1 scoop disengage protein
- 1 tablespoon flax seeds
- 1/2 cup ice cubes

Instructions:
1. Put all of the parts directly into the blender or food processor. Mix until

smooth.

Serves: 2

Prep. Time: 3 minutes

Blend Time: 2 minutes

Dietetic Facts

Serving Size: 233 g

Calories: 124 Total

Fat: 2.6 g

Saturated Fat: 0 g Trans. Fat: 0 g

Cholesterol: 0 mg

Sodium: 99 mg

Potassium: 200 mg

Total Carbohydrates: 12.4 g Dietary

Fiber: 2.5 g Sugar: 9.4 g

Protein: 25.3 g

Almond Strawberry Fruit Drink

—————T

his crunchy adaptation is loaded with protein and mixes the delectable flavors and has heart-solid supplements, which makes it an incredible without dairy Fruit Drink. This drink is refreshingly nutty and smooth. **Ingredients:**

- 16 ounces unsweetened Almond milk
- 8 almonds
- 2 enormous strawberry, frozen
- 1 1/2 scoop whey protein powder or 3 tablespoon gelatin
- 6 ice cubes

Instructions:

Put all of the parts solidly into the blender or food processor.

Blend until smooth.
Serves: 2
Prep. Time: 3 minutes
Blend Time: 2 minutes
Dietetic Facts
Serving Size: 272 g
Calories: 162 Total
Fat: 5.7 g
Saturated Fat: 0 g Trans. Fat: 0 g
Cholesterol: 0 mg
Sodium: 218 mg
Potassium: 230 mg
Total Carbohydrates: 3.8 g
Dietary Fiber: 1.8 g Sugar: 0.8 g
Protein: 26 g
Vitamin A: 0% Vitamin C: 12%
Calcium: 30% **Iron:** 7%

Chocolate Avocado Cream Fruit Drink

T

he avocado in this Fruit Drink makes for a corruptly flavorful beverage. Rich, smooth, and smooth. The avocado additionally loads this beverage with a sound measure of good fats.

Ingredients:
- 1 avocado, frozen
- 1/2 cup weighty cream
- 1 tablespoons dull chocolate
- 1 teaspoon Splenda
- 1 pack gelatin or 1 scoop chocolate detach protein
- 1 cup water

Instructions:
1. Put all of the parts solidly into the blender or food processor. Mix until

smooth

Serves: 2
Prep. Time: 3 minutes
Blend Time: 2 minutes
Dietetic Facts
Serving Size: 286
g Calories: 450
Total Fat: 32.3 g
Saturated Fat: 12.1 g Trans. Fat: 0 g
Cholesterol: 42 mg
Sodium: 53 mg
Potassium: 535 mg
Total Carbohydrates: 16.6 g Dietary
Fiber: 6.9 g Sugar: 7.2 g Protein:
26.9 g
Vitamin A: 12% Vitamin C: 17%
Calcium: 6% **Iron:** 6%

Very Berry Strawberry Fruit Drink

he mysterious to a thick cold Fruit Drink is utilizing frozen foods grown

Tfrom the ground frozen milk. This drink is stacked with flavors and nutrients and is best served on a warm summer day.

Ingredients:
- 2 ounces Greek yogurt, strawberry
- 1/4 cup berries, frozen
- 1/2 cup unsweetened almond milk
- 1 teaspoon Splenda
- 1 pack gelatin or 1 scoop seclude protein

Instructions:
Put all of the parts directly into the blender or food processor.

Blend until smooth.
Serves: 1
Prep. Time: 3 minutes
Blend Time: 2 minutes
Dietetic Facts
Serving Size: 249
g Calories: 197
Total Fat: 2 g
Saturated Fat: 1 g Trans. Fat: 0 g
Cholesterol: 3 mg
Sodium: 163 mg
Potassium: 224 mg
Total Carbohydrates: 11.5 g Dietary
Fiber: 1.8 g Sugar: 8.8 g
Protein: 30.4 g
Vitamin A: 0% Vitamin C: 13%
Calcium: 23% **Iron:** 5%

Peach Coconut Fruit Drink

resh summer peaches and coconut milk make this a sweet, rich without
F

dairy mix. Utilizing chilled coconut milk gives it a milkshake-like consistency. The coconut milk additionally makes it additional rich and velvety with

the high amount of healthy fats.

Ingredients:

- 1 1/2 peaches, frozen
- 1 cup coconut milk
- 1 tsp. lemon zest
- 2 pack gelatin
- 1 cup ice

Instructions:

1. Put all of the parts solidly into the blender or food processor. Mix until smooth.
Serves: 2
Prep. Time: 3 minutes
Blend Time: 2 minutes
Dietetic Facts
Serving Size: 342 g
Calories: 399 Total
Fat: 28.8 g
Saturated Fat: 25.4 g Trans. Fat: 0 g
Cholesterol: 0 mg
Sodium: 76 mg
Potassium: 464 mg
Total Carbohydrates: 13.9 g
Dietary Fiber: 3.8 g Sugar: 10.2 g
Protein: 27.4 g
Vitamin A: 5% Vitamin C: 16%
Calcium: 4% **Iron:** 14%

Coconut-Strawberry Fruit Drink

W

ith only 5 fixings, this sans dairy Fruit Drink is rich and sweet. The vanilla makes this mix taste like frozen yogurt. I love to add a tad of unsweetened destroyed coconut subsequent to mixing for added flavor.

Ingredients:

- 5 strawberries, frozen
- 1 cup unsweetened coconut milk
- 1 tablespoon ground flax seed
- 1 pack gelatin or 1 scoop seclude protein
- 1 teaspoon vanilla extract

Instructions:

Put all of the parts solidly into the blender or food processor.

Blend until smooth.

Serves: 1
Prep. Time: 3 minutes
Blend Time: 2 minutes
Dietetic Facts
Serving Size: 219
g Calories: 438
Total Fat: 31 g
Saturated Fat: 25.7 g Trans. Fat: 0 g
Cholesterol: 0 mg
Sodium: 76 mg
Potassium: 475 mg
Total Carbohydrates: 13.8 g Dietary
Fiber: 5.7 g Sugar: 7.6 g
Protein: 28.4 g
Vitamin A: 0% Vitamin C: 64%
Calcium: 5% **Iron:** 25%

Cocoa-Coconut-Macadamia Fruit Drink

I

f you haven't tried creamy, crunchy macadamia nuts, then it's about time you do! These nuts are high in heart-healthy omega 3 fatty acids, which are also important for the nervous system and fights inflammation.

Ingredients:
- 1 ounce (2 tbsp.) ground macadamia nuts
- 3/4 cup unsweetened almond milk
- 1 tablespoon unsweetened cocoa powder
- 2 teaspoons Splenda
- 1/2 teaspoon vanilla extract
- 1 g salt
- 2 pack gelatin
- 1 cup ice cubes

Instructions:
1. Put all of the parts solidly into the blender or food processor. Mix until smooth.

Serves: 2
Prep. Time: 3 minutes
Blend Time: 2 minutes
Dietetic Facts
Serving Size: 236 g
Calories: 240 Total
Fat: 12.4 g
Saturated Fat: 2.1 g Trans. Fat: 0 g
Cholesterol: 0 mg
Sodium: 321 mg
Potassium: 172 mg
Total Carbohydrates: 8.3 g
Dietary Fiber: 2.5 g Sugar: 4.8 g
Protein: 26 g

Vitamin A: 0% **Vitamin C:** 0%
Calcium: 15% Iron: 8%

Chocolate-Coconut Tofu Fruit Drink

T

his high fat, high protein Fruit Drink possesses a flavor like a chocolate milkshake. The tofu makes this organic product drink smooth, practically like pudding. This drink is a yummy method for beginning the day! **Ingredients:**

- 80 ml unsweetened coconut milk
- 1/2 cup tofu, silken
- 1 tablespoon unsweetened cocoa powder
- 150 ml water
- 1 teaspoon Splenda
- 1 pack gelatin or 1 scoop segregate protein

Instructions:

1. Put all of the parts squarely into the blender or food processor. Mix

until smooth.

Serves: 1
Prep. Time: 3 minutes
Blend Time: 2 minutes
Dietetic Facts
Serving Size: 395 g
Calories: 401 Total
Fat: 25.4 g
Saturated Fat: 18.7 g Trans. Fat: 0 g
Cholesterol: 0 mg
Sodium: 88 mg
Potassium: 488 mg
Total Carbohydrates: 13.6 g Dietary
Fiber: 4.7 g Sugar: 7.6 g
Protein: 37.2 g
Vitamin A: 0% **Vitamin C:** 4%
Calcium: 29% Iron: 25%

Almond Chocolate Blueberry Fruit Drink

———————T

his mix is as nearly as rich tasting and smooth as an exemplary milkshake, just this rendition is low carb! The blueberries and cocoa powder help the cell reinforcement properties of this Fruit Drink. **Ingredients:**

- 1 cup unsweetened almond milk
- 1/4 cup blueberries, frozen
- 1/4 tsp vanilla extract
- 1 tablespoon unsweetened cocoa powder
- 1 teaspoon Splenda
- 1 pack gelatin or 1 scoop disconnect protein

Instructions:

1. Put all of the parts directly into the blender or food processor. Mix until

smooth.

Serves: 1
Prep. Time: 3 minutes
Blend Time: 2 minutes
Dietetic Facts
Serving Size: 324 g
Calories: 185 Total
Fat: 4.4 g
Saturated Fat: 0.8 g Trans. Fat: 0 g
Cholesterol: 0 mg
Sodium: 236 mg
Potassium: 306 mg
Total Carbohydrates: 13.3 g Dietary
Fiber: 3.7 g Sugar: 6.8 g
Protein: 26.3 g
Vitamin A: 0% Vitamin C: 10%
Calcium: 32% Iron: 13%

Just Peachy Fruit Drinks

———T

his mix is an invigorating, solid Fruit Drink that is loaded with protein. When in season, I love to substitute the blueberries with a peach for an adjustment of shading and flavor.

Ingredients:

- 1 1/2 cups peaches, frozen
- 6 ounces Greek yogurt
- 1 cup diminished fatt milk
- 4 pack gelatin
- 1 cup ice

Instructions:

Put all of the parts directly into the blender or food processor.

Blend until smooth.

Serves: 4

Prep. Time: 3 minutes

Blend Time: 2 minutes

Dietetic Facts

Serving Size: 255 g

Calories: 181 Total

Fat: 2.3 g

Saturated Fat: 1.4 g Trans. Fat: 0 g

Cholesterol: 7 mg

Sodium: 99 mg

Potassium: 221 mg

Total Carbohydrates: 10.8 g Dietary

Fiber: 1 g Sugar: 9.8 g

Protein: 30.8 g

Vitamin A: 5% **Vitamin C:** 7%

Calcium: 14% Iron: 3%

Apricot Fruit Drink

T̶h̶i̶s̶ Fruit Drink is not difficult to make and just requires 5 fixings. It has
T

the ideal measure of sweet-tart flavor and the entire milk and Greek yogurt improves the yummy apricot flavor. The additional protein makes this treat

feel more like a meal.

Ingredients:
- 6 ounces Greek yogurt
- 1 cup entire milk
- 1 1/2 cups apricot
- 4 pack gelatin or 4 scoops disengage protein
- 1 cup ice

Instructions:
1. Put all of the parts directly into the blender or food processor. Mix until

smooth.

Serves: 4
Prep. Time: 3 minutes
Blend Time: 2 minutes
Dietetic Facts
Serving Size: 248 g
Calories: 276 Total
Fat: 9.3 g
Saturated Fat: 8.7 g Trans. Fat: 0 g
Cholesterol: 3 mg
Sodium: 104 mg
Potassium: 311 mg
Total Carbohydrates: 11.1 g Dietary
Fiber: 1.1 g Sugar: 10 g
Protein: 31.0 g
Vitamin A: 25% Vitamin C: 11%

Calcium: 14% **Iron:** 3%

Apricot Peachy Slush

———————W

hen you need something cold to drink, nothing tastes better compared to a frosty natural product drink! Attempt this smooth mix of peach and apricot for a reviving beverage that is high in Vitamin C.

Ingredients:
- 5 1/2 ounces apricot nectar
- 2 peaches
- 1 1/2 cups ice
- 1 tablespoon lemon juice
- 1 1/2 cups carbonated water

Instructions:

Put all of the parts directly into the blender or food processor.

Blend until smooth.

Serves: 4

Prep. Time: 3 minutes

Blend Time: 2 minutes

Dietetic Facts

Serving Size: 270g

Calories: 42 Total

Fat: 0.2 g

Saturated Fat: 0 g Trans. Fat: 0 g

Cholesterol: 0 mg

Sodium: 5 mg

Potassium: 2143 mg

Total Carbohydrates: 10.4 g Dietary

Fiber: 1 g Sugar: 4.2 g

Protein: 0.6 g

Vitamin A: 13% Vitamin C: 44%

Calcium: 2% **Iron:** 2%

Conclusion

T hank you again for downloading this book. I trust that the plans assist you with remaining on the Ketogenic Diet!

www.ingramcontent.com/pod-product-compliance
Lightning Source LLC
Chambersburg PA
CBHW080629030426
42336CB00018B/3130